1

Fruit Infused Water Recipes

Disclaimer

No part of this article can be transmitted or reproduced in any form including print, electronic, photocopying, scanning, mechanical or recording without prior written permission from the author.

While the author has taken utmost efforts to ensure the accuracy of the written content, all readers are advised to follow information mentioned here at their own risk. The author cannot be held responsible for any personal or commercial damage caused by misinterpretation of information.

All information, ideas and guidelines presented here are for educational purposes only and readers are encouraged to seek professional advice when needed.

Summary

Spa treatments are a great way to relieve stress and have a wonderful time. They help relax the body and refresh you, so that you come out feeling energized. However, what do you do when you simply can't go to the spa for relaxation? Well, the answer is simple. You can create those treatments at home without much work.

Now I know what you must be thinking. A spa treatment at home without much work, is that even possible? The answer is: Yes! Not only is it possible, you can also create all kinds of aroma that are used in spa treatments, so you can pamper yourself whenever you feel like it. This book is especially written for people who want to bring the spa to their homes.

Fruit Infused Spa Water has been created for the purpose of helping you get the experience of a relaxing and calming feel from the comfort of your own home. This book is a goldmine for people who want to rehydrate and maybe put a finishing touch to a home spa experience whenever they want. It contains information on the various health benefits you can obtain through fruit infused spa water.

Along with this, it consists of 50 recipes that will simply blow you away. These 50 recipes have been prepared just for this book, and will give you an idea of how to make fruit infused spa water in your home.

So without further ado, start reading this book, and surprise your friends and family with a spa experience in your very home. Are you ready to get started on this exciting adventure?

Then let us begin!

Contents

What is Fruit Infused Spa Water

Coming home after a tiring day at work, soaking yourself in warm water infused with herbal extracts is so relaxing. With soothing water like that waiting for you at home, you would want to rush home every day. But what if the nutrients and aroma of fruits could also be gained from the water? Wouldn't that be simply wonderful?

You must be thinking that this is only possible when you go for a spa treatment. Well, little did you know, you can create the same water and ambiance right in the confines of your home. It is very easy and so relaxing that you would want to do this every day. And guess what? You can even drink the fruit infused spa water making it simply amazing to have this deliciously soothing drink at home.

All you need are the right ingredients and you are set up for creating different variations of fruit infused spa waters. Add them in the bath to make it more luxurious, or simply have them all day long to remain hydrated with a flavorful punch. Drinking water can seem quite tedious, particularly when you are one of those people who simply forget to stay hydrated. Infusing fruits in water is a great way to add some flavor to it, making you want to drink more and more.

In this book, we will discuss the different benefits of using fruit infused spa waters and then include a variety of recipes, so that you may enjoy homemade spa water. Make sure to follow the instructions as provided in the book, and always let the fruits infuse according to the proper guidelines.

Benefits of Fruit Infused Spa Water

Having enough water on a daily basis is crucial for the proper functioning of the body. Every cell in the body functions with the help of water, which makes it imperative to drink as much water as possible. Fruit infused water helps in increasing the daily consumption of water, making it much easier and tastier to consume greater amounts. Not only that when this water is created for the purposes of using it as spa water it provides many benefits which helps in rejuvenating your body and giving it the lift it needs after a tiring day.

Following are the benefits you can gain through Fruit Infused Spa water.

1. It helps in helping you control your appetite, while providing you the hydration you require to remain energized and function properly throughout the day.
2. Along with this, when fruit infused water is taken orally it helps in strengthening the immune system of the body, while preventing heartburn, regulating the sugar level of the blood, helping you in managing and maintaining your weight.
3. Green tea mixed with lime is an excellent combination for soothing the headaches, and freshens up your breath. Not only that most fruit infused waters help in improving the digestive system of the body, and helps in supporting the fat burning process.
4. You can also gain many beauty benefits from fruit infused spa water. It is known to improve the texture of the skin, along with appearance.
5. It also helps in regulating the PH levels of the skin, and helping it remain hydrated for longer periods.
6. Fruit infused spa water provides a good dose of Vitamin C to the skin, and helps the kidney maintain its health.
7. This water is exceptionally beneficial for it provides the necessary support required to fight cancer.

Infusing different ingredients will help you in gaining different benefits. Following is the list of ingredients along with the various advantages they offer.

1. Green Tea, Lime and Mint, when infused together in water, help in burning the fat, aid digestion, reduce headaches, improve congestion, all the while acting as a breath freshener.
2. Strawberry when combined with Kiwi and water results in the improvement of cardiovascular health, protection of the immune system, regulation of the blood sugar level, and digestion.
3. Cucumber, Lemon, Lime and Water when mixed together, and infused overnight, help in managing the weight, reduction in bloating, controlling the appetite, increasing hydration levels of the body, and digestion woes.

4. Lemon, Orange, water, and Lime, helps in improving the Digestive system of the body, while providing vitamin C, strengthening immune defense, and decreasing heartburn (if it is taken at room temperature).

5. Lemon, water, and Ginger Root, when soaked in water overnight results in healthier skin, improving digestion, and cleansing of the liver with all impurities.

Let us immediately begin looking at the vast array of recipes you can use to create fruit infused spa water in your home.

Fruit Infused Spa Water Recipes

1. Mint, Strawberry, Lemon and Water Detox

Makes about 2 Liters

This spa water is exceptionally delicious with the scent and taste of strawberries, while it is packed full of nutrients and mineral that are unique only to strawberries and lemon. It helps in eliminating all the toxins from the body that will help you become fit and healthy.

Ingredients

Water, about 6-8 cups

2 cups of ice cubes

5 mint leaves

15 strawberries, quartered

1 thinly sliced lemon

Method

Take a large pitcher. Proceed to fill it with water while make sure that it is not filled to the brim. Add in the rest of the ingredients, except the ice and the mint leaves. Add in the mint leaves after squeezing them slightly without tearing them apart, so that the oils can be released. You can choose to put in the ice cubes before, or after all of the ingredients have been soaked in water. However, it may be best to put them in after the other ingredients have been added. Let all the ingredients infuse in the water for at least an hour before serving it. Leaving it in the fridge overnight is far more effective.

Once you have started consuming it, and the water level reduces to 1/4th the height of the pitcher, then refill it with water and add in ice cubes as required.

2. Delicious Cucumber and Lemon Water

Makes about 2 Liters

This spa water is loaded with nutrients and minerals that are essential for the body. The vitamins gained from this water will give plenty of energy in your body while causing an anti-inflammatory effect. This helps in reducing the acidity of heartburn that is felt after fatty food intake. Apart from this, it also helps in boosting the immunity system of the body.

Ingredients

Water, about 6-8 cups

2 cups of ice cubes

¼ cucumber, finely sliced

½ lemon, finely sliced

Method

Fill a large pitcher with water and then add all of the ingredients in it, making sure to add the ice cubes last. Let them soak overnight and then drink it the next day. Refill the pitcher with water when only 1/4th of it is left in the pitcher. Keep it refrigerated at all times.

3. Day Spa Apple Cinnamon Water

Makes about 2 Liters

This Spa Water is very beneficial for the body, as cinnamon acts as a sugar controller, and apple is packed full of iron, traces of which are infused in the water and transmitted to the body as it is consumed. It helps in fighting off stomach infections, while ensuring that you remain hydrated throughout the day.

Ingredients

1 whole apple, thinly sliced

2 cups Ice cubes

1 whole cinnamon stick, broken in half

Water

Method

Combine all of the ingredients in a pitcher full of water, and add in the ice cubes last. Let the ingredients soak in the water for 12-24 hours, and then drink it the entire day. If you are short on time, then you can also refrigerate it for at least an hour, before serving.

4. Mango Ginger Spa Water

Makes about 4 Liters

This Spa water gives you the benefit of ginger, mixed with the flavor of mango. Ginger is very beneficial as it helps in fighting off acidity and gastroenteritis, and helps in improving your digestion. Mango provides nutrients your body requires to remain energized and healthy.

Ingredients

I inch ginger, peeled and thinly sliced

1-cup mango, chopped and frozen

Water

Ice cubes

Method

Cut the ginger into 3-4 slices, about the size of a small coin. Add them in a pitcher filled with water and then add in the mango pieces. Add in the ice cubes next, and let them soak overnight or for an hour, if you are in a hurry. Drink it all day long, and then refill it 2-3 times or until the water loses the flavor of the ingredients.

5. Orange Ginger Spa Water

Makes about 1 Liter

Orange is one of the most delicious fruits rich in Vitamin C. When infused with water, not only does it add flavor to the water, but it also infuses its own properties to the water. Ginger is a good anti-inflammatory ingredient, which helps in easing any knots or stress in the stomach and improves digestion. When these two are combined and infused together in water, they help in improving the acidity level of the body, and help maintain it at optimal level.

Ingredients

1-cup ice cubes

1 inch of ginger, chopped

1 orange, segmented

Water, about 3-4 cups

Method

Peel the ginger and then slice it into thick slices, then add them in the pitcher. Top it with the orange followed by the ice cubes. Fill the pitcher up to the brim with water and let this concoction refrigerate for an hour. Best results can be obtained if the ingredients are soaked in the water overnight. Drink this for the rest of the day and enjoy the nourishing freshness it provides. Refill it with water until the ingredients lose their flavor.

6. Tangerine and Strawberry Infused Spa Water

Makes about 2 Liters

This Spa water is exceptionally beneficial for the skin. After drinking this water continuously for a couple of days, you will see a significant difference in your. It will be smoother, healthier, and more radiant.

Ingredients

Water, about 6-8 cups

2 cups ice cubes

1 tangerine's rinds; make sure to remove the white pith entirely

½ cup strawberries, dried or fresh, and quartered

Method

Place the tangerine in a large teapot or kettle and then add in the strawberries, followed by the water, then let the water come to a boil. Once it is boiled, let the ingredients infuse in the water for an hour while it cools, then pour the water through a sieve to remove any fruit debris or fruit and then pour in a glass, add the ice cubes and enjoy!

Note: Make sure that the water is enough to fill a large pitcher, and then add in as many ice cubes as desired.

Makes about 2 Liters

This water is delicious as the lime adds a zing to it, while the strawberry adds a hint of sweetness to the water. Drinking it will help you in getting rid your body's harmful minerals and toxins. Not only that, it also helps in speeding up the process of digestion, thereby, making it easier for the essential nutrients to get absorbed quickly.

Ingredients

Water, about 6-8 cups

2 cups ice cubes

1 lime, thinly sliced

8 strawberries, quartered, fresh or frozen

Method

Combine the strawberries and lime in the pitcher followed by the ice cubes, and the pour in the water. Let the ingredients remain soaked in the water for 3-4 hours before serving. Best results can be obtained if left overnight in the refrigerator, then simply pour in a glass, and enjoy this heavenly concoction. Refill the pitcher with water at least 2-3 times, or until the flavor disappears.

8. Fall Fruit Infused Spa Water

Makes about 2 Liters

This Spa water is packed full of fall fruits. It is bursting with the vitamins, minerals and nutrients your body needs. The water also helps in providing your body four organic acids that act as digestive enzymes that help in improving digestion. Along with this, it also helps in getting rid of the fatty deposits that are stuck within the liver and the lymphatic system.

Ingredients

1 tsp. all spice berries,

Water, about 6-8 cups

2-3 cups ice cubes

1 tbsp. cranberries, dried

1 orange, sliced into 8ths

1 pear, thinly sliced

Method

Add all of the ingredients in a pitcher full of water then add in the ice cubes and let the ingredients infuse with the water overnight. Drink this concoction the next day, and enjoy! Refill the pitcher with water at least 2-3 times or until the flavor of the fruits is lost.

9. Watermelon, and Rosemary Infused Spa Water

Makes about 2 Liters

This water contains high amounts of nutrients, vitamins, and minerals that are essential for the body. It also contains antioxidants, which are infused and obtained through the watermelon. Rosemary is also known for its ability to prevent some of the major diseases like cancer, and even acts as a pain relief and mood elevator. When these two ingredients are combined and infused in water, you will immediately feel relaxed and in a better mood.

Ingredients

Water, about 6-8 cups

1 large sprig of rosemary

2-3 cups of ice cubes

2 cups watermelon, chopped into small cubes

Method

Add all of the ingredients in a pitcher full of water and then add in the ice cubes to help the ingredients remain submerged in the water. Once you are done, place the pitcher in the refrigerator. This mixture should be refrigerated for 3-4 hours, at the very least, and if possible, overnight. Drink this concoction the next day, making sure to refill it, when the water level reduces to 1/4th of the original mixture.

10.   Cucumber Citrus Water

Makes about   2 Liters

Cucumber and citrus is a great combination, which works very well in improving the overall health of the body. After drinking this water your skin will feel healthier, and you will notice that it glows more.

Ingredients

Water, about 6-8 cups, (about half a gallon or more)

1 large cucumber, finely sliced

1 large orange, finely sliced

1 large lime, finely sliced

1 large lemon, finely sliced,

2-3 cups of ice cubes

Method

Add all of the fruits in a large pitcher, followed by the ice cubes, and then pour in the water in it. Once done, let the ingredients soak in the water for 3-4 hours or overnight, for better flavor. Enjoy this delectable drink all day long. When the water in the pitcher is about to finish make sure to add in more, and refill it 2-3 times or until there is no more flavor left.

11. Minty Orange Spa Water

Makes about 2 Liters

Mint and orange is a great combination, as it helps you in overcoming gastroenteritis, and other problems related to the stomach. After drinking this water, you will feel lighter and more energetic. It helps in breaking up the harmful fats in the body, and helps in slimming you down, while remaining fit

Ingredients

Water, about 6-8 cups

10 mint leaves

2-3 cups of ice cubes

3 large oranges, sliced

Method

Add all of the ingredients in a large pitcher filled with water then add in the ice cubes and refrigerate for an hour or overnight, if possible. Serve and enjoy this delicious fruit infused spa water with your friends and family. Make sure to refill the water as it is consumed, until the flavor of the fruits is lost.

Makes about 2 Liters

This water is exceptionally beneficial and tasty. It helps in fighting off the signs of aging while boosts bone development. You will feel stronger once you have consumed this water. It also hydrates you faster than normal water, as cucumbers are known for their ability to hydrate the body.

Ingredients

Water about 6-8 cups

¼ cantaloupe, chopped into small dices

2-3 cups of ice cubes

¼ honeydew melon, chopped into small dices

1 large cucumber, finely sliced

Method

Add all of the ingredients in a large pitcher, followed by the ice cubes, and then pour the water in, until it is filled to the brim. Once done, place the pitcher in a refrigerator and let the water refrigerate overnight, for best results. Drink this concoction the next day, and then refill the pitcher with water when it reaches 1/4th its height. Make sure to refill it at least 2-3 times or until the infused water loses its flavor. Enjoy with your friends and family.

13. Watermelon Basil Spa Water

Makes about 2 Liters

This Spa water is healthy for the body, as it is packed full of nutrients, while remaining pleasing to the taste buds. After the flavors and nutrients of the watermelon are infused in the water, you will feel refreshed and rejuvenated, along with energized for the rest of the day.

Ingredients

Water, about 6-8 cups

12 basil leaves, washed

2-3 cups of ice cubes

2 cups watermelon, seedless, and chopped into small cubes

Method

Add all of the ingredients in a large pitcher and then add in the ice cubes. Pour the water until it reaches the brim, and then let the ingredients soak in it for at least 4 hours or overnight. Pour in a glass and drink the whole day, making sure to refill the pitcher every time the water is consumed.

Makes about 2 Liters

This Spa Water is simply delicious, as it consists of the freshness of coriander and nutrients of citrus fruits. As these fruits are rich in Vitamin C, you can be sure to remain hydrated while drinking this flavorful water. Drinking this water helps in preventing different kinds of skin disorders, so be sure to drink plenty of water throughout the day.

Ingredients

Water, about 6-8 cups

¼ cup leave of cilantro

1 large orange, thinly sliced

1 large lime, thinly sliced

1 large lemon, thinly sliced

Method

Add all of the ingredients in a large pitcher filled with water, making sure to add in the ice cubes last and then place the pitcher in the fridge to refrigerate for 3 hours or overnight if possible. Drink this concoction for 24 hours, making sure to refill the pitcher with water when the water level reaches 1/3rd of its height, or until the flavor of the fruits is lost. Enjoy with your friends and family.

15.   Lavender and Lemon Spa Water

Makes about 2 Liters

Lavender always adds spectacular fragrance and flavor to any food, and when it's flavor is combined with the tanginess of lemon, you will have a spectacular Spa Water experience. The water helps in relaxing your nerves, and serves as a great mood improver. Drink this water and feel relieved, see the difference in your skin, as it will improve the more you drink this Spa Water.

Ingredients

½ a gallon of water

2-3 cups of ice cubes

¼ cup fresh lavender

3 lemon, large and cut in thick slices

Method

Add all of the ingredients in a large pitcher filled with water. Add in the ice cubes last and then place the pitcher in the refrigerator and let the ingredients soak for more than 4 hours. It is best to let them soak overnight. Drink this concoction the next day, making sure to refill the pitcher with water until the flavor is lost.

16.   Honeydew and Lime Spa Water

Makes about 2 Liters

Honeydew is packed full of flavor, vitamins, and nutrients. When steeped in water, part of its nutrients is infused with the water. Drink this water to improve your metabolism, along with strengthening your immune system.

Ingredients

Water, about 6-8 cups

4 sprigs of mint, rinsed and washed

1 lime, sliced in thick round slices

2-3 cups of ice cubes

2-3 slices of honeydew melon; make sure that it is ripe

Method

Take a large pitcher and one by one, add all of the ingredients in it, making sure to add in the ice cubes last. Pour water in the pitcher on top of the ingredients. Refrigerate this concoction overnight and then drink it the next day, making sure to refill it as required. Enjoy it with your friends and family.

Makes about 2 Liters

Berries are always a treat to have, and when infused in water, the water takes on a charm, which is unique only to berries. Add rosemary to it, and you get a sweet and mouthwatering aroma. Drink this delicious Spa Water and have your body feel stronger and lighter, all the while getting healthier.

Ingredients

Water, about 6-8 cups

2 fresh sprigs of rosemary, above 4 inches long

2-3 cups of ice cubes

1-cup blueberries, fresh

Method

Lightly crush the blueberries and the rosemary, to help release more flavor, and then add them in a large pitcher. Add in the ice cubes next, and then fill the pitcher with water, let the ingredients soak in it, overnight or for 4 hours, until the flavor has infused into the water, then enjoy this drink for the entire day, making sure to refill it until the water loses its flavor.

Makes about 2 Liters

This Spa Water is very beneficial for you as it contains nutrients from different fruits. Feel energized after having this water, and experience improvement in the overall health of your body. The water also consists of vitamins that are essential for the body, and helps in boosting its immune system.

Ingredients

Water, about 6-8 cups

2 cups apples, chopped and frozen

2 cups grapes, frozen

2 cups berries, frozen

2-3 cups ice cubes

Method

Add all of the ingredients into a large pitcher, with the ice cubes going in last, and then fill it with water, then place it in the fridge to refrigerate for a couple of hours, or overnight of possible. Enjoy this refreshing drink with your friends and family, and make sure to refill the pitcher with water until the flavor is lost.

Makes about 2 Liters

Strawberries are not only delicious but also extremely beneficial for the body. They contain some of the most essential nutrients, which are required for the body to function properly. Drink plenty of water to remain hydrated during the day, while reaping the benefits this tasty water offers.

Ingredients

Water, about 6-8 cups

½ cucumber, cut into fine slices

2-3 cps of ice cubes

4 strawberries, sliced

Method

Add the cucumber slices and strawberries in a pitcher filled with water, then add in the ice cubes. Refrigerate this overnight and drink the next day to feel rejuvenated.

20. Pineapple Strawberry Fusion Spa Water

Makes about 2 Liters

Pineapple and strawberries is a brilliant combination of two ingredients, which complement one another. This Spa Water helps in rejuvenating your body, and is exceptionally beneficial for your skin. After drinking this yummy water, your skin will become clearer, and more radiant. A natural glow will appear on your skin, as it becomes healthier.

Ingredients

Water, about 6-8 cups

One carton of strawberries, quartered

2-3 cups of ice cubes

One whole pineapple, peeled, cored and sliced

Method

Add the pineapple and strawberries in a large pitcher, and then add the ice followed by pouring water over it. Refrigerate the pitcher. Let the concoction chill for at least 3 hours, giving the ingredients time to soak in the water. Refrigerate overnight, if possible. Drink this refreshing water the entire day, making sure to refill the pitcher until the flavor of the ingredients is lost.

Makes about 2 Liters

This Spa Water is so smooth in texture that you can't help but enjoy it. It contains many nutrients, which help the body in improving its overall health. Make sure to drink plenty of water to keep yourself hydrated. This water also helps in improving your immune system.

Ingredients

Water, about 6-8 cups

1 vanilla bean, sliced along the length and the seeds scraped from it

2 peaches, pitted and peeled, then quartered

2-3 cups of ice cubes

Method

Add the vanilla bean and peaches in a large pitcher filled with water, and then add the ice followed by pouring water in. Refrigerate the pitcher allowing the ingredients to soak and infused their flavor with the water for a couple of hours. Best results are obtained if refrigerated overnight. Drink this water when it's ready, and feel refreshed with every sip. Refill the pitcher as the water level reaches 1/3rd of its height. Keep refilling until the flavor is lost.

Makes about 2 Liters

This Spa Water is simply divine, and the benefits it has to offer will blow you away. Not only does it help in cutting down the harmful fats and converting them into energy for the body, it also helps in slimming down the body while providing essential nutrients. Stay hydrated by drinking this flavorful water and feel energized throughout the day.

Ingredients

Water, about 6-8 cups

2 cups pineapple slices, fresh

2-3 sprigs of mint

2-3 cups of ice cubes

Method

Add in all of the ingredients in a pitcher and then fill it with water. Let the ingredients soak in it, for at least 4 hours, or overnight, if possible. You can drink this delicious fruit infused spa water the entire day. You will feel refreshed and hydrated the entire day. Refill the pitcher as the water level goes down, or until the flavor of the fruits is lost. Enjoy this refreshing drink with your friends and family.

23.   Strawberry and Kiwi Infused Spa Water

Makes about 2 Liters

This Spa Water is simply delicious, with the flavors of strawberry and Kiwi infused in it. It is packed full of nutrients and vitamins, so make sure to drink it. After drinking this water you will feel refreshed and energized, as it helps you in staying fit and healthy.

Ingredients

Water, about 6-8 cups

2 cups strawberry, quartered

1-cup kiwi, sliced

2-3 cups of ice cubes

Method

Add in all of the ingredients in a pitcher and then fill it with water. Refrigerate the concoction overnight to get best results, and then drink this concoction all day, all the while refilling the pitcher with water until the flavor is lost. Make sure to let the ingredients remain soaked in it for as long as possible, for better infusion. Enjoy with your friends and family.

Makes about 2 Liters

This Spa Water is chock full of flavor and nutrients. You will get a flavorful surprise when you drink this water, and feel stronger. This is mainly because of the vitamins and minerals that are present in the water. Keep yourself hydrated by drinking this spa water throughout the day and feel rejuvenated.

Ingredients

Water, about 6-8 cups

Teavana Strawberry Lemonade Herbal Tea

4-5 Bay Leaves

2-3 cups of ice cubes

2 lemons, sliced thinly

10 strawberries, large and quartered

Method

Boil water, enough to fill the pitcher and then let the tea steep in it for a couple of minutes, (around 3-4 minutes). Allow the water to cool before adding in the rest of the ingredients, with the ice added last, and then place it in the fridge for 3 hours. Once chilled, enjoy this concoction with your friends and family. You can refill it with water until the flavor is lost or simply enjoy it as is.

Makes about 2 Liters

This Spa Water is so delicious that you will want more. Not only that, it is extremely beneficial as this water helps in restoring the body to a healthy state while helps in fighting off the signs of aging. It also helps in improving your skin and makes it healthier.

Ingredients

1 cucumber, small and sliced thinly

Water, about 6-8 cups

1 lemon, thinly sliced

2 peaches, cored, peeled, and quartered

2 cups ice cubes

Method

Add all of the ingredients in a large pitcher filled with water, and let it refrigerate overnight or for a minimum of 4 hours. Drink this concoction all day to keep you hydrated and refreshed. Keep refilling the pitcher with water until the flavor is lost.

Makes about 2 Liters

This Spa Water has the combined properties of apples, strawberries, and mint. What does this mean? It means, that drinking this water will boost your metabolism and immune system, while providing you energy by breaking down the saturated fats in your body.

Ingredients

Water, about 6-8 cups

1 apple, cored and chopped into small pieces

2 cups ice cubes

1-cup strawberry, quartered

8-12 mint leaves, fresh and washed

Method

Add all of the ingredients in a pitcher filled with water, and let them soak overnight until the flavor is deeply infused with it. Drink this spa infused water all day, making sure to refill it as the water is consumed. Enjoy this with your friends and family.

Makes about 2 Liters

Drink this Spa Water for a clear and healthy skin. It will help eliminate all toxins from your body, while ensuring that your body receives all of the essential nutrients, which will improve its overall health. Make sure to drink plenty of water and keep yourself hydrated, so that you may remain hydrated at all times.

Ingredients

Water, about 6-8 cups

Lemon, finely sliced

2 sprigs of rosemary

Berries of your choice

2 cups ice cubes

Method

Add the lemon, rosemary and berries in a pitcher filled with water and then add the ice cubes. Refrigerating the concoction for a couple of hours or overnight, if possible, will help the infusion process. Don't forget to drink this yummy concoction the next day, while refilling the pitcher until the flavor of the fruits is lost. Enjoy this super delicious and refreshing fruit infused spa water with your friends and family.

28. Berry, Ginger and Mint Spa Water

Makes about 2 Liters

This Spa water is not only delicious but also healthy. It is anti-inflammatory, as it consists of ginger, which is one of the best anti-inflammatory ingredients and helps in reducing acidity in the body.

Ingredients

Water, about 6-8 cups

1 tbsp freshly grated ginger

2 cups raspberries, frozen

1 cup blackberry, frozen

2 cups ice cubes

½ lemon, sliced thinly

A handful of mint

Method

Add all of the ingredients in a large pitcher filled with water, and then pour the ice on tops then add the water in. Place the pitcher in a fridge for a couple of hours, or overnight. Drink this water the entire day. It will leave you feeling refreshed and energized throughout the whole day. Make sure to refill the pitcher with water as the water level reaches 1/4th of its height. Enjoy it with your friends and family.

Makes about   2 Liters

This Spa Water is packed full of nutrients and minerals that are required by the body to remain healthy and fit. Drinking it in large amounts can help the body improve its digestive system, while ensuring that it keeps the body fit. It also helps in preventing inflammations, and other digestive problems within the body.

Ingredients

Water, about 6-8 cups

 2 sprigs of Rosemary, fresh

2 sprigs of Mint, fresh

2 cups ice cubes

½ lemon, thinly sliced

½ cucumber, thinly sliced

2-3 strawberries, quartered

Method

Add all of the ingredients in a pitcher filled with water, making sure to add the ice last. Then allow the ingredients to soak in water for 5 hours, or overnight, if possible. Drink this refreshing fruit infused spa water, and serve it to your friends and family. Refill the pitcher when the water level in it decreases, and keep refilling until the flavor of the herbs and fruits is lost.

30.   Blueberry Coconut Spa Water

Makes about   2 Liters

This Water is delicious and helps the body in remaining healthy. It helps you in getting rid of the harmful toxins, and fats. Along with this, it provides the body with energy and strength.

Ingredients

3 cups coconut water

Water, as required, for filling the pitcher

1 cup blueberries, slightly mashed to bring out the flavor

2-3 cups ice cubes

Method

Add all of the ingredients in a large pitcher, followed by the water, enough to fill it to the brim, and then refrigerate it overnight. Enjoy it the next day, and keep refilling the pitcher until the flavor is lost.

Makes about 2 Liters

This Spa Water is very beneficial for the body as it consists of Vitamins and Minerals, which are essential for the body. It also helps in improving and strengthening the immune system.

Ingredients

Water, about 6-8 cups

10 mint leaves

6 Meyer lemon's zest, seeds removed, and finely sliced

3-4 cups ice cubes

Method

Add all of the ingredients in a large pitcher filled with water, and then refrigerate it for at least 6 hours, or overnight, if possible. Once done, drink this concoction for the whole day, adding water every time it's about to be finished, or until the flavor is lost.

32.   Apple, Rosemary, and Pomegranate Spa Water

Makes about   2 Liters

This Spa Water is packed full of nutrients and consist of Vitamins and Minerals, which help in boosting the metabolism of the body. Drink this water in large quantities, and feel refreshed and energized. It helps in improving the overall health of the body, by providing required nutrients.

Ingredients

Water, about 6-8 cups

35 pomegranate seeds

The Juice of 2 lemons

10 apples, cored and thinly sliced

½ cup rosemary, fresh

2 cups ice cubes

Method

Add all of the ingredients in a large pitcher, followed by the ice cubes, and then fill the pitcher with water. Let these ingredients soak for 24 hours, while refrigerated. Then enjoy this delicious fruit infused spa water the entire day, and keep refilling it until the water loses its flavor.

Makes about   2 Liters

This Spa Water is so delicious and tasty that you will keep coming back for more. Along with this it has the taste of pear and the benefits of ginger, which make it a good option to have for keeping yourself hydrated. Have plenty of this water, and have your mood improve as your health improves.

Ingredients

Water, about 6-8 cups

½ cup ginger, freshly peeled and chopped into fine thin slices

10 pears, cored and chopped into small pieces

2-3 cups of ice cubes

Method

Place all of the ingredients in a pitcher filled with water, and then refrigerate it for a couple of hours, or overnight. Enjoy this concoction the next day, and drink it as much as possible, all the while adding more water in the pitcher as the water level in it reduces. Keep at it until the flavor is lost.

34.   Fennel, Tangerine, Apple, and Thyme Spa Water

Makes about   2 Liters

This Spa Water is packed full of flavor, and consists of many nutrients which helps energizing you and keeping your body healthy. It is quite tasty, and improves the digestive system, thereby, making it easier for you to digest food.

Ingredients

Water, about 6-8 cups

2 fennel bulbs, shaved

2 sprigs of thyme

2 cups ice cubes

12 tangerine zests, and fruit, with their pith removed

Method

Add all of the ingredients in a pitcher filled with water, and then refrigerate this concoction for 5 hours, or overnight, if possible. Drink this water the entire day, after the ingredients have soaked in it, and then refill the pitcher until the flavor is lost.

35. Agaus Frescas Spa Water

Makes about   2 Liters

Ingredients

Water, about 6-8 cups

½ cantaloupe, chopped into small pieces

1 cucumber, large and finely sliced

2 cups ice cubes

½ honeydew melon, chopped into small pieces

Method

Add all of the ingredients in a pitcher filled with water, and let them soak in it for a couple of hours, or overnight for best results, and then drink it the entire day, making sure to refill it until the flavor is lost. Enjoy with your friends and family.

Makes about   2 Liters

This Spa Water is all about the Southern Charm. After drinking this water, you will feel energized, and happy. It helps in improving the mood, while ensuring that your body's immune system improves.

Ingredients

Water, about 6-8 cups

1 tsp. salt

2 cups strawberries, quartered

4 cups watermelon, sliced with seeds removed

2-3 cups ice cubes

Method

Add all of the ingredients in a large pitcher filled with water, adding the ice cubes at the last, and then refrigerate it for 6 hours or overnight. Drink this fruit infused spa water the entire day, refilling it every time it is consumed, until the water loses the fruit's flavor.

Makes about 2 Liters

This Spa Water is definitely a crowd pleaser. You will feel rejuvenated and fresh after drinking this water, and it will also help you in overcoming any overweight issues. You can remain fit and healthy while drinking this water, and reap all the benefits it has to offer.

Ingredients

Water, about 6-8 cups

2 oranges, peeled and segmented

1 cucumber, small and thinly sliced

2 limes, thinly sliced

2 lemon, thinly sliced

2-3 cups of ice cubes

Method

Place all of the ingredients in a large pitcher, adding the ice cubes last, and then fill it to the brim with water. Let the ingredients soak for a couple of hours or overnight for best results, then drink this concoction the next day. Make sure to refill it about 6-8 cups until the flavor of the fruits is lost. Enjoy this delicious fruit infused spa water with your friends and family.

38. Mint, Orange and Lemon Medley

Makes about   2 Liters

This Spa Water is delicious and contains Vitamin C, which helps in preventing different diseases. Make sure to drink plenty of this water to remain healthy, smart, and hydrated at all times.

Ingredients

Water, about 6-8 cups

8 mint leaves

1 orange, thinly sliced

2 cups ice cubes

1 lemon, thinly sliced

Method

Add all of the ingredients in a pitcher filled with water, and allow the ingredients to soak for a couple of hours, Enjoy this drink the entire day, and keep adding in more water until the flavor of the fruits is lost.

Makes about   2 Liters

This Spa Water is delicious and packed full of nutrients. It helps in boosting your immune system, along with improving the digestive system. Make sure to drink this water throughout the day to keep yourself hydrated.

Ingredients

Water, about 6-8 cups

½ cup mint leaves, fresh

1 cantaloupe, peeled, deseeded and cut into small pieces

2-3 cups of ice cubes

1 cup watermelon, chopped into small pieces

½ Honeydew melon, chopped into small pieces

Method

Add all of the ingredients in a pitcher filled with water, and then allow them to soak for 6 hours. Drink this concoction during the day, and feel refreshed. Add more water as the spa water is consumed, until the flavor of the fruits is lost.

40. Orange and Pineapple Spa Water

Makes about   2 Liters

This Spa Water consists of Vitamin C and the flavors of Orange and Pineapple are simply amazing. It helps in getting rid of the toxins from the body, and also helps in improving the functioning capability of the liver. This improves your body's ability to get rid of any harmful materials, and strengthens your immune system.

Ingredients

Water, about 6-8 cups

½ orange, thinly sliced

½ pineapple, fresh and thinly sliced

2-3 cups of ice cubes

½ inch ginger, finely sliced

Method

Add all of the ingredients in a pitcher filled with water and then refrigerate this concoction overnight to allow the fruits flavor to infuse in the water. Drink this water the entire day, and keep refilling it until the flavor is lost.

Makes about   2 Liters

This Spa Water is quite delicious and consists of the nutrients that make the body stronger and more agile. It helps provide energy to the body, thereby keeping your focused and sharp throughout the day.

Ingredients

Water, about 6-8 cups

2 oranges, finely sliced

Cranberries, a handful

2 cups of ice cubes

2 sprigs of rosemary

1 apple, cored and thinly sliced

Method

Add all of the ingredients in a large pitcher, with the ice cubes added at the end, and then fill it to the brim with water. Let the ingredients soak for the couple of hours, during which refrigerate this concoction. Enjoy this spectacular fruit infused water, and refill it as it reaches 1/4th of its height, until the flavor of the fruits is lost.

Makes about   2 Liters

Drinking this Spa Water will help improve your digestive system, by providing the nutrients which help in improving the overall functions of the body. It also helps in improving blood circulation, and helps you remain focused and energized throughout the day.

Ingredients

Water about 6-8 cups

The juice of one blood orange

2 cups ice cubes

1 vanilla bean, cut lengthwise

Method

Place all of the ingredients in a large pitcher filled with water, and let the ingredients soak in it for 5 hours. Refrigerate it during this time, and then enjoy this drink with your friends and family. Make sure to refill it until the flavor of the fruit is lost.

Makes about   2 Liters

This Spa Water is packed full of flavor and nutrition, and is very healthy for the body. It's delicious taste allows you to consume more water that will keep you hydrated. You will also feel relaxed and content, as his water helps in improving mood.

Ingredients

5-6 mint leaves

Water, about 6-8 cups

½ orange, finely sliced

Ginger, very finely chopped, a healthy pinch

2-3 cups ice cubes

Vanilla beans, sliced lengthwise, with the pods removed and added

Method

Add all of the ingredients in a large pitcher filled with water and then refrigerate it for a couple of hours. Drink this water the entire day, making sure to add in additional water, until the flavor is lost. Enjoy this drink with your friends and family.

Makes about   2 Liters

This Spa Water has the nutrition of watermelon, the sour and sweet flavor from the lime, and a hint of freshness from mint. Once you drink it, you would want to have more. It helps in improving the overall functions of the body, while ensuring that you remain energized and healthy.

Ingredients

Water, about 6-8 cups

12 sprigs of mint,

4 thin slices of lime

6 tbsp. lime Juice, freshly squeezed

3 cups watermelon, ½ inch cubes

2-3 cups ice cubes

Method

Add all of the ingredients in a large pitcher filled with water, and allow the ingredients to soak for a couple of hours, about 4. Refrigerate during this time, and then enjoy this refreshing water during the day, adding more water in the pitcher as it is consumed, until the flavor is lost.

Makes about   2 Liters

This Spa Water is what you need during the day to keep yourself hydrated while making sure that your body remains healthy and fit. It helps in strengthening the body against external agents, such as viruses by strengthening the immune system.

Ingredients

Water, about 6-8 cups

2 cups Watermelon, chopped into small cubes

1 lemon, finely sliced

2 cups ice cubes

Method

Add all of the ingredients in a pitcher filled with water, and then let then soak while refrigerating for7 hours. Drink this water regularly, refilling it with more water as it is consumed, until the flavor of the fruits is lost.

Makes about   2 Liters

This Mojito is packed full of flavor and all of the essential vitamins and minerals. Try it out and feel the difference for yourself. Your skin will feel radiant, the texture of your hair will improve, and you will feel refreshed after every sip.

Ingredients

Water, about 6-8 cups

1 box of blueberries

Key limes, thinly sliced

6 mint leaves, fresh

2 cups ice cubes

Method

Add all of the ingredients in a large pitcher, adding the ice cubes last, and then fill it to the brim with water. Refrigerate it overnight, and then enjoy this delicious drink, while refilling it every time it reaches 1/4th of its height, until the flavor of the fruits is lost.

47. Kiwi, Blueberries, and Lemon Spa Water

Makes about   2 Liters

This Spa Water is a great combination of Kiwi, Blueberries, and Lemon. You can be sure to enjoy your day while drinking this water and keeping yourself hydrated. Make sure that you drink this water, for it is exceptionally beneficial for the heart and protects you from various diseases.

Ingredients

2 Kiwi, thinly sliced

1-cup blueberries

Water, about 6-8 cups

1 lemon, thinly sliced

2 cups ice cubes

Method

Add all of the ingredients in a large pitcher filled with water, and then refrigerate it for 6 hours or overnight to allow the ingredients to soak and infuse with the water. Drink this yummy water for the whole day, all the while adding in more water as it is consumed, until the flavor is lost.

48.   Mango, Watermelon Spa Water

Makes about   2 Liters

Drinking this Spa Water will not only provide you energy, but also help you in remaining fit and active throughout the day. Try out this water and see the difference in yourself.

Ingredients

1 cup mango, chopped into small cubes

Water, about 6-8 cups

1 cup watermelon, chopped into small cubes

2 cups ice cubes

Method

Add all of the ingredients in a large pitcher filled with water, and then refrigerate it overnight. Drink this water for the entire day, making sure to refill it until the flavor is lost.

Makes about   2 Liters

This Spa Water has the combined flavors of orange, mango, and pineapple. Drinking this water will help you in getting rid of any toxins, while ensuring that your immune system remains strong.

Ingredients

Water, about 6-8 cups

1 cup pineapple, chopped into small cubes

1 orange, thinly sliced

1 cup mango, chopped into small dices

2 cups ice cubes

Method

Place all of the ingredients in a large pitcher filled with water, and then refrigerate it overnight, is possible, or for at least a couple of hours. Enjoy this rejuvenating drink the next day, refilling it every time it is consumed, until the flavor of the fruits is lost.

50.   Blueberry, Mint, and Mango Spa Water

Makes about   2 Liters

Being packed full of nutrition, this Spa Water is a great way to spend the day. It keeps you hydrated and helps in improving the digestive systems, thereby, reducing any chances of getting an upset stomach. Enjoy this Spa Water during the day, and obtain a glowing and radiant skin.

Ingredients

Water, about 6-8 cups

1-cup blueberry

4-5 sprigs of mint, fresh

1-cup mango, chopped

2-3 cups ice cubes

Method

Add all of the ingredients in a large pitcher filled with water, refrigerating it overnight to allow the flavors to infuse well together. Drink this concoction the next day, all the while refilling it, until the flavor is lost.

Delicious Spa Water – Created

Drinking this delicious water will not only leave you wanting more, but also help you in staying energized while remaining hydrated at all times. This is one of the best methods of reminding yourself to drink, particularly during hot weather, as you will simply love the taste of the fruits, which have been infused in it.

Make sure that you follow the recipes exactly as they have been mentioned in the book, so that you may have an enjoyable and relaxing time throughout your day. Also, you can add this to your bath, with a sweet fragrant aroma, mix it with a little bit of lavender oil, and salt, and voila, you have created a spa treatment in your very home.

The fruity flavor adds more flavorful choices to the everyday simple water, and helps you stay alert and hydrated. With the sun getting warmer by the minute, Fruit Infused Spa Water is just what you need to rejuvenate yourself throughout the day. Drink lots and stay hydrated.

So what are you waiting for? Browse through this book, gather the ingredients, soak them in water, and start drinking!